Contents

M000074564

CHLORELLA VULGARIS

AND

CHLORELLA VULGARIS EXTRACT (CVE)

The Powerful Japanese Medicinal Green Algae as a Biological Response Modifier

Toshihiro Kanno, Ph.D.

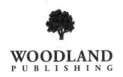

WOODLAND
P U B L I S H I N G

Copyright © 2005 by Toshihiro Kanno, Ph.D.
All rights reserved. No part of this publication may be reproduced, stored in a
retrieval system, or transmitted in any form without the prior written permis-
sion of the copyright owner.

For order information or other inquiries, please contact us:
Woodland Publishing
448 East 800 North
Orem, Utah
84097
Visit us at our Web site: www.woodlandpublishing.com
or call us toll-free: (800) 777-2665

The information in this book is for educational purposes only and is not recommended as a means of diagnosing or treating an illness. All matters concerning
physical and mental health should be supervised by a health practitioner knowl-
edgeable in treating that particular condition. Neither the publisher nor the
author directly or indirectly dispenses medical advice, nor do they prescribe any
remedies or assume any responsibility for those who choose to treat themselves.

ISBN 1-58054-403-7
Printed in the United States of America

Foreword

Our world has changed dramatically in the last few decades: global industrialization and the explosion of the human population have led to the rapid extinction of many species, the pollution of earth and water and a decrease in joy, zest and vitality in the western population. Depression, chronic fatigue, neurological disorders—especially in children—chronic degenerative diseases and many other forms of slow decline are steadily on the rise. Conventional Medicine has conquered life threatening acute illnesses but is almost helpless in the face of chronic disease and the consequences of the ever increasing body burden of toxins. Breast milk of nursing moms—the most sacred of all foods—is polluted with flame retardants. Our brains harbor more and more heavy metals. Our immune system is fighting the onslaught of ever increasing amounts of man-made environmental toxins. Even the most remote streams in the Himalayas are polluted now with mercury. Not many people have genetically determined perfect detoxification enzymes. Many of us do not make enough glutathione-S-transferases or have blocked liver detoxification pathways.

But we are not doomed. Nature has provided us with the most perfect protection from it all: chlorella. This true algae is millions of years old, has been through a lot in its evolution and has prepared itself to be our perfect rescue food. Chlorella is about the size of a red blood cell and has a polysaccharide membrane that can absorb large amounts of dioxin, lead, mercury and other toxins. On the inside of the cell are the true miracles:

- Protein: chlorella contains roughly 50 percent protein and aminoacids (ideal nutrient for vegetarians), Vitamin B6, minerals, chlorophyll, beta carotene and more
- Methyl-cobolamine, the most absorbable form of Vitamin B12 (food for the nervous system, restores damaged neurons and has ist own detoxifying effect)
- Sporopollein is as effective as cholestyramin in binding neurotoxins and more effective in binding toxic metals then any other natural substance found.
- Lipids (12.4 percent) alpha-and gamma-linoleic acid help to balance the increased intake of fish oil recommended for prevention of neurodegenerative diseases and are necessary for a multitude of functions, including formation of the peroxisomes.
- CVE (*Chlorella vulgaris* extract) helps the body detoxify also. A recent in-vivo study shows the rapid and successful removal of lead from toxic lab animals
- The porphyrins in chlorophyl have their own strong metal binding effect. Chlorophyll also activates the receptor on the nucleus of the cell which is responsible for the formation of the peroxisomes, the cell organelles which are responsible for detoxification.

Studies have shown chlorella also to remove dioxin and other carcinogens from the body in a very gentle and yet effective way. I have used chlorella as a major food staple for myself and my clients for many years. The results are very obvious: babies, whose moms have consumed chlorella during the pregnancy are healthier and smarter. Many people have successfully recovered from neurological damage and disease. People stay younger and fitter. Japanese business men use chlorella to prevent hangovers and flues. I have used chlorella also for chronic pain and joint problems and to protect patients from toxicity if they are exposed in their work environment. But foremost, I use it as a source of good healthy vegetarian protein that is easily digested and absorbed by most. Chlorella is the ideal survival food for the coming challenges in human evolution. Chlorella is as natural and pure as it gets. Why not add it to your diet or your nutritional program? It makes good sense.

This booklet presents a small selection of the vast available literature and should serve as encouragement for those of you who consider a more natural approach to life and well-being.

Dietrich Klinghardt, M.D., Ph.D.

Dietrich Klinghardt specializes in using biological detoxification in the treatment of chronic illness. He lectures worldwide on the principles of Applied Neurobiology and is the director of the American Academy of Neural Therapy. His neurotoxin elimination protocol has helped people all over the world to regain vitality and health.

Preface

Your local health-food store features a wealth of supplements, all promoted as necessary to good health. But people who are trying to improve their well-being or have specific physical conditions can't help but wonder, "What do these products really do?" and "Which ones are right for me?" Unfortunately, some supplements are sold with wild promises, even though their effects are not proven.

This booklet will introduce you to the benefits of a health-food supplement called CK-strain chlorella. Chlorella is a type of green algae, and CK-strain chlorella is the most intensively studied variety of chlorella. ("CK-strain" is an abbreviation for "Chlorella Kougyo-Strain.") This booklet outlines the research data showing why CK-strain chlorella is a vital health-promoting addition to any diet.

Introduction

So many of us eat without really thinking about what we're putting in our bodies. This is unfortunate, because diet is fundamental to human health. (In fact, the Chinese character for "food" means "bettering humans.") But a good diet depends on choosing what to eat and how much to eat; otherwise, food can actually harm us.

In Japan, for example, people's food choices have changed significantly in recent years. Because the Japanese diet is becoming more like the American and European diet, various diseases associated with the Western diet are increasing in Japan.

Figure 1A: Annual transition of food intake

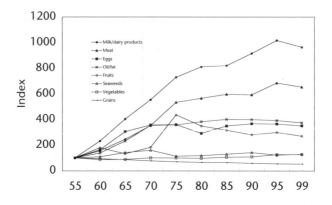

Figure 1B: Annual transition of patients' visits

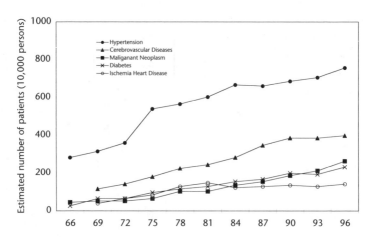

According to a nationwide Japanese nutrition survey, the average diet is significantly different from that of 1955, when the diet was well-balanced (Figure 1A). The intake of dairy products is 10 times higher than before; meat products, seven times higher; and the intake of eggs and fats is four times higher. Consumption of animal products has increased significantly, and vegetable and grain intake hasn't changed much. The new Japanese diet is high in protein and fat and low in fiber, just like the Western diet.

These dietary changes have caused an increase in body fat, viscous (or sticky) blood, and damaged blood vessel walls and a rise in dietary-related diseases such as hypertension, diabetes, hyperlipemia, cancer, heart disease, and cerebrovascular diseases (Figure 1B). These diseases are rampant in Western countries. In the United States, the number one cause of death is heart disease. The main cause of death in many advanced countries is related to diet.

Chlorella is one of the best health-food supplements for the prevention and cure of diseases that are caused by diet. Let's examine why.

Living things develop their body structures by eating food during the process of evolution, starting with simple single-celled organisms. When living things eat food, they must have systems that can identify whether the food is safe or harmful, and systems that can eliminate harmful substances from their bodies. The physical structure of an organism's metabolic, nervous, and immune systems has been developed by eating food during the process of evolution.

Chlorella is a type of algae, which is the very origin of the food chain and is the food that contributed to building the physical structures of living things, including humans, during evolution. Thus chlorella is a highly regarded health-food supplement for maintaining the human body.

Chlorella was introduced to the health-food marketplace about 40 years ago. In 1964, commercial cultivation of chlorella was established in Japan, and today Japan, Korea, Taiwan, and Indonesia produce chlorella. It is used not only for health-food supplements, but also in processed foods, food additives, medication additives, marine feeds, feed additives, and fertilizers.

Chlorella is helpful for supplementing nutrients of high-quality, plant-based proteins, vitamins, minerals, chlorophyll, and antioxidants. Chlorella can help lower cholesterol, regulate the intestines, detoxify the body, lower blood pressure, and regulate the immune system. Chlorella helps the human body maintain balance.

For these reasons, chlorella is one of the best health-food supplements for the prevention and improvement of diseases caused by poor diet. This booklet focuses on CK-strain chlorella, which is the most effective variety.

What Is Chlorella ?

Chlorella likely appeared on Earth 1.5 to 2 billion years ago. It is a fresh-water, one-celled green algae that is widely found in lakes and marshes all over the world. The name chlorella is a compound of Greek (chloros, meaning green) and Latin (ella, meaning small thing), and it was discovered and named by M.W. Beyerinck of Holland in 1890.

Chlorella is 2 to 10 microns in size (slightly smaller than a red blood cell), and with an optical microscope you can see its green and almost spherical shape. It's classified botanically in the division of chlorophyta, the class chlorophyceae, order chlorococcales, family of oocystaceae, and genus of chlorella. It's an ancestor of such vegetables as spinach and pumpkins.

Compared to other plants, chlorella has a high concentration of chlorophyll, so its capability for photosynthesis is many times higher than that of other plants. Photosynthesis is the process by which green plants synthesize nutrients such as starch out of water and carbon dioxide by absorbing energy from the sun. Chlorella also has a compound called chlorella extract that is capable of multiplying cells into four parts every 20 hours. This impressive cell-multiplication capability is unique to chlorella and is rarely seen in other living things.

Chlorella helps maintain human health and prevent and treat disease because of its high-quality, plant-based protein, vitamins, minerals, dietary fiber, antioxidant compounds, and chlorella extract.

CK-strain Chlorella

Not all chlorella has the same compounds and capabilities. Chlorella has evolved since it first appeared, and now it's classified into groups with different characteristics. Chlorella is separated into species according to the shape of the cells, the shape of the chlorophyll, and other variables. There are 20 to 30 species, such as *Chlorella vulgaris*, *Chlorella pyrenoidosa*, and *Chlorella ellipsoidea*. The species are also differentiated into groups called strains. Even though these strains are the same chlorella species, they may have different capabilities.

When we use chlorella for health-food supplements, the compounds, characteristics, and physiological activities of the product are significantly different according to the species or strain. This is especially true for health-food supplements, and the type of chlorella strain makes a tremendous difference in the value of the supplement you buy.

Chlorella vulgaris CK-strain is the strain that provides the most benefits for human health.

Benefits of *Chlorella vulgaris* CK-strain are as follows:
• Supplements various nutrients such as proteins, vitamins, minerals, dietary fibers, and antioxidant compounds
• Aids absorption and digestion of food
• Thinner cell wall (its cell wall is 1/5th to 1/10th the thickness of other strains of chlorella)
• 82 percent digestion/absorption rate
• Secretes polysaccharide around the cell
• The stickiness of the CK-strain is part of the active ingredient, called CVE (*Chlorella vulgaris* extract)
• Its compounds help recover weakened resistance and physical strength
• Scientific proof of effectiveness
• More than 500 scientific research reports have been published proving chlorella's safety and effectiveness
• More than 90 percent of research conducted worldwide on chlorella focuses on CK-strain chlorella

The polysaccharide secreted around the cells of CK-strain is *Chlorella vulgaris* extract (CVE). When CK-strain is stained red and observed through an electron microscope, the stained polysaccharide layer around the cell can be seen (Figure 2). If it's a general type of chlorella, polysaccharide around the cell is not observed, even with the red stain. It's noteworthy that CK-strain secretes polysaccharide around its cell.

Among chlorella products, there is an extract called CGF (chlorella growth factor). This name comes from chlorella extract research in 1960 that showed the acceleration of cell division and growth when chlorella extract was administered to microorganisms such as lactobacilli and yeast. But growth promotion is only one of many beneficial characteristics of chlorella extract. This booklet will focus on the CK-strain chlorella extract, CVE, which has been studied extensively.

CVE, one of the active compounds of CK-strain, has been found to boost the immune system, improve metabolism, improve liver function, lower blood pressure, and lower blood sugar.

Figure 2: CK-Strain Chlorella

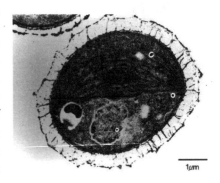

1μm

When CK-Strain is stained with ruthenium red, the stained polysaccharide layer around the cell can be observed through an electron microscope. Common chlorella do not show this extra cellular polysaccharide even with the same stain. A notable characteristic of CK-Strain is to secrete polysaccharide around its cell.

CK-strain also has extremely thin cell walls (Figure 3A). A cell wall of CK-strain is about 20nm thick. By comparison, the cell walls of chlorella ellipsoidea C-87 are 110-210 nm, *Chlorella vulgaris* C-30: 50 nm, chlorella fusca var. vacuolata 211/8p: 120 nm, and chlorella vulgaris C-209: 200 nm. These other strains are five to 10 times thicker than CK-strain (Figure 3B). The thickness of the cell wall makes a big difference in the digestion and absorption of the nutrient when it's processed into health-food supplements.

For 40 years, researchers have tested water all over the world to find high-quality chlorella. So far, no one has found chlorella that outshines CK-strain chlorella.

Digestibility of Chlorella

Most strains of chlorella have thick cell walls and are considered hard to digest. However, a 1977 report explained that when the cell wall of chlorella was broken, the digestibility improved[1]. Because of this report, many chlorella products with broken cell walls were distributed. Even today, there are many chlorella products sold based on this data.

In 1996, the National Consumer Affairs Center of Japan conducted tests on chlorella products and reported on the quality, sanitary grade, and legitimacy of cell wall breakage. The report stated, "Cell wall breakage does not make a difference in digestibility of chlorella." Using the CK-strain, Komaki and others[2] researched whether cell wall breakage is necessary for improving digestibility. Komaki prepared CK-strain with the cell walls broken and with no treatment, comparing the artificial digestion rate (a method measuring how much protein is disintegrated in a certain time period after putting CK-strain and digestive enzymes into test tubes) and the digestion/absorption rate in small animals. The results showed no difference. The tests also indicated that cell wall breakage was not necessary in order to improve digestibility.

The digestibility of chlorella depends on the strain of chlorella used. Because CK-strain chlorella has an extremely thin cell wall, it can be digested very well without breaking its cell wall. The Japan Food Hygiene Association tested the digestion/absorption rate and

Figure 3: Electron Microscope Pictures of Chlorella

(A) Chlorella vulgaris CK-strain   (B) Common Chlorella vulgaris

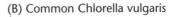
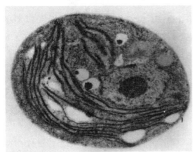
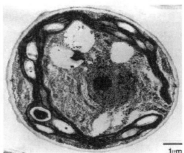

(A) Electron microscopic picture of Chlorella Vulgaris CK-Strain. They show that CK-Strain has a thin cell wall.The thickness is about 20nm and digestibility absorption rate is 82%.
(B) Electron microscopic picture of a common chlorella vulgaris cell. Common chlorella has a thick cell wall and its thickness is 100 to 200nm. It's 5 to 10 times thicker than CK-Strain.

found the rate with small animals was 82 percent (Test Certification No.T034-00305), indicating its digestibility was excellent.

Some chlorella with thicker cell walls is sold by promising that the digestibility is improved by breaking the cell wall. However, there are very few products that clearly describe what percent of the chlorella cell is broken, or how much the digestibility is improved. Furthermore, chlorella's original characteristics and physiological effects do not change by breaking the cell. Rather, the cell-wall breaking process may degrade the quality of protein and may cause the disintegration of vitamins and fats (including unsaturated fatty acids) and oxidation. When you are choosing a chlorella supplement, you should make sure the product is scientifically proven, regardless of the advertisement.

How CK-strain Helps Prevent Diseases Caused by Poor Diet

Diseases such as hyperlipemia, hypertension, diabetes, arteriosclerosis, heart disease, stroke, and cancer are closely related to diet. Heredity; aging, with its lowered resistance; and environmental factors such as chemical substances and stress are also linked to these ailments.

These diseases are on the rise in advanced countries. Heart disease, stroke, and cancer are the most prevalent causes of death in many countries.

In order to prevent these diet-related illnesses, we must regulate and balance the diet, along with improving lowered immune function and protecting the body from health-threatening chemical substances and stress.

Scientists have proven that CK-strain is effective for balancing the diet; improving lowered cell function and resistance; and detoxifying chemicals and alleviating stress. CK-strain chlorella can help prevent and treat many diet-related diseases.

How CK-strain Chlorella Can Help the Everyday Diet

Each food we eat has a certain effect. Meat and fish are rich in protein and help build the body's structure. Carbohydrate foods, or staple foods, such as bread, rice, potatoes, and pasta, are rich in sugar and are converted to both instant energy and stored energy. Vegetables and fruits are rich in vitamins, minerals, dietary fiber, and antioxidants that help the other foods do their jobs; in other words, they are the body's regulators.

Since each food plays its own role in the body, the correct amount to eat of each is of vital importance. Dr. Kawashima, the former chief of the Food Industry Research Center and professor at Oubirin University, proposed that what and how much to eat should be determined by the number and shape of the teeth. Humans have four canine teeth for chewing meat; eight incisor teeth for crunching vegetables and fruits; and 20 molar and premolar teeth for grinding staple foods. In a simple ratio, meat is one, vegetables are two, and staple foods are five. This is the well-balanced ratio for eating.

The typical diet today is far from well-balanced. Vegetables, which regulate the body, are especially lacking in most diets. For that reason, meat dishes and staple foods cannot do their jobs and remain in the body as fat, so that improperly metabolized food causes disease.

This unbalanced diet means food becomes body fat. Increased body fat results in hyperlipemia (high cholesterol and triglycerides), not only clogging the blood with fat, but also raising the risk of diabetes, hypertension, and arteriosclerosis.

As shown in Table 1, CK-strain chlorella effectively supplies the body with nutrients that are identical to those found in vegetables.

1. LOWERING OF CHOLESTEROL IN THE BLOOD AND LIVER

Eating is one of life's joys. It's a human instinct to want to eat a lot of delicious food, and this desire influences our lives. But eating

Table 1: Nutritional Profile

Protein	60.39 g	Lipid	9.89 g
Non fibrous		Dietary fiber	
carbohydrates	6.51 g	(Prosky method)	13.5 g
Chlorella extract	24.9 g	Chlorophyll	2700 mg
Total carotenoid	180 mg	Vitamin B1	2.33 mg
Niacin	30.2 mg	Pantothenic acid	2.10 mg
Vitamin B2	5.18 mg	Vitamin B6	0.54 mg
Vitamin B12	190 µg	Folic acid	26.9 µg
Biotin	73.3 µg	Choline	270 mg
Inositol	270 mg	Vitamin C	4 mg
Ergosterol		Vitamin E	8.9 mg
(Provitamin D2)	90 mg	Vitamine K1	2600 µg
Linoleic acid	2.31 g	Linolenic acid	1.50 g
Iron	120 mg	Magnesium	300 mg
Calcium	130 mg	Potassium	1100 mg
Zinc	1300 µg	Copper	280 µg
Manganese	4300 µg	Chromium	28 µg
Cobalt	410 µg		

JAPAN INSTITUTE OF OILS & FATS, OTHER FOODS INSPECTION
Analysis certificate No.01-0101

an unbalanced diet increases excessive body fat and can lead to various diseases. It is well known that increased body fat promotes the secretion of certain oxidants from lipocytes.

The substances that disturb insulin (tumor necrosis factor-alpha, or TNF-α), raise blood pressure, clog the blood, and promote arteriosclerosis are secreted by fat cells when the body's fat increases. Accumulation of body fat results in high cholesterol and triglycerides and raises the risk of hypertension, diabetes, and arteriosclerosis. For those who are already at risk for these diseases, the threat increases.

Along with balancing the diet, CK-strain chlorella cleans the blood by eliminating excess fat and making the blood vessels more flexible. Numerous studies have confirmed that CK-strain chlorella can help ailments caused by an unbalanced diet and help purify the blood.

When CK-strain chlorella is given to test animals who have been fed high-cholesterol food, the value of serum and liver cholesterol decreases. If high-cholesterol food is given first, the excessive cholesterol is stored in the body. When the animals are then given CK-strain chlorella, it lowers the value of serum and liver cholesterol significantly by promoting the excretion of the stored cholesterol[3]. In tests with hyperlipemia patients4, serum cholesterol and LDL-cholesterol were substantially lowered after administering 9 g of CK-strain chlorella for one year (Figure 4). CK-strain chlorella works to lower cholesterol by suppressing the absorption of bile acids and cholesterol in the intestines and promoting the excretion of bile acids and cholesterol into feces.

These studies show that CK-strain aids in the excretion of blood cholesterol and liver cholesterol and helps cleanse the blood.

2. IMPROVEMENT OF HYPERTENSION

According to the American Public Health Service, 50 million people in the United States have hypertension, and more than 50 percent of people over 65 are affected. Men tend to suffer hypertension and high blood pressure more than women, but women reach the same risk level after menopause.

Hypertension is often called the "silent killer" because there are no symptoms until it becomes a problem. The blood vessels and

Figure 4: CK-strain for low cholesterol in hyperipemia patients

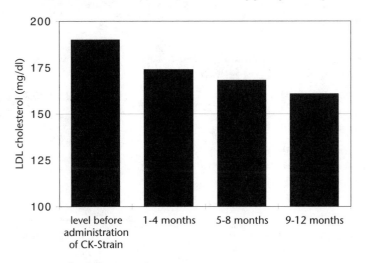

heart become overburdened without warning, and strokes and heart attacks can occur suddenly.

CK-strain chlorella was tested on rats with spontaneous hypertension (SHR) and prevented their blood pressures from rising[5,6] (Figure 5A). When CK-strain chlorella was given to 15 hypertension patients over 60 years of age for seven to eight years, all of them experienced lower blood pressure[7] (Figure 5B). There was a 20-30 percent decrease in systolic blood pressure and a 20-25 percent decrease in diastolic blood pressure. The values of lipid metabolism, cholesterol, β-lipoprotein, triglycerides, urine Na/K ratio, and urine K/N ratio also improved, bringing them close to normal levels.

CK-strain chlorella helps lower blood pressure by dilating the blood vessels with minerals, such as potassium and magnesium; nuclear acid substances, such as adenosine; amino acids, such as cysteine and glycine; and CVE.

3. IMPROVEMENT OF DIABETES

Diabetes affects 125 million people worldwide, and the number is increasing every year. According to the World Health Organization, the number is expected to increase to 300 million by 2025. Diabetes has indeed become a global pandemic.

Diabetes is basically high blood sugar due to insulin deficiency. This deficiency happens when the pancreas doesn't secrete enough insulin to process sugar properly, a problem called insulin resistance. This means the blood sugar doesn't get into the cells easily and is not readily used as energy, triggering complications such as retinopathy, nephropathy, neurosis, hypertension, arteriosclerosis, and infectious diseases.

Deterioration of the insulin function is caused by heredity

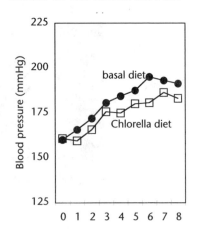

Figure 5A: Antihypertensive effect of CK-strain on rats

Figure 5B: Antihypertensive effect of CK-strain on patients

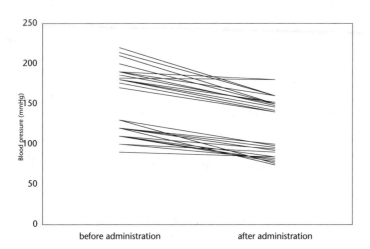

and/or the wrong diet. Research has shown that CK-strain can correct an unbalanced diet and support insulin function, helping to prevent and lessen the effects of diabetes.

A. Improvement in regimen. The basic treatment for diabetes is diet therapy. However, it's hard to maintain for many people. It's also easy to overlook deficiencies of micronutrients and difficult to supplement "green nutrients" such as vitamins, minerals, and dietary fibers, so food supplements become necessary.

A number of studies have looked at the effect of introducing CK-strain chlorella to the diabetic diet[8].

In one study, CK-strain chlorella was administered to eight diabetic patients ranging from 50 to 80 years of age every day in order to improve their nutrition. Four were taking oral blood-sugar suppressants. By using CK-strain chlorella for diet therapy, body weight, fasting blood pressure, and total cholesterol could be controlled, bringing them closer to normal levels. Three of the four patients taking the blood-sugar suppressants didn't need them anymore. This study proved that CK-strain chlorella can help manage and control diabetes.

The effects of CK-strain chlorella on diet therapy for patients who have complications of diabetes have also been examined[9].

CK-strain chlorella was given to 18 patients who had complications due to diabetes (five had diabetic retinopathy, six had diabetic neuropathy, four had diabetic nephropathy, and three had arteriosclerosis obliterans) in order to improve the nutrient balance of their diets. Compared to a group not using the chlorella, the test group improved their conditions by about 1.7 times, proving that CK-strain chlorella helps lessen complications due to diabetes when introduced to the diet.

B. Improvement in metabolism. Diabetes results in an inefficient use of glucose, depriving the body of energy. In order to make up the difference, muscle tissue decomposes, and the resulting amino acids are used as an energy source. Muscle decomposition aggravates symptoms, and the concentration of serum amino acids becomes very high compared to that of healthy people. Phenylalanine, leucine, and isoleucine are especially increased, since they are more difficult to use for energy. Thus diabetes triggers not only the abnormality of sugar metabolism but also of protein metabolism. This protein decomposition, called protein dysbolism, causes radical weight loss as diabetes worsens.

Studies have been done on CK-strain chlorella's effect on protein dysbolism caused by diabetes[10].

The serum amino acids of patients who were given insulin (over 10 units per day) showed high levels of all amino acids after one year (an increase of 10 to 15 percent), despite the insulin treatment. It's clear that insulin treatment alone does not improve protein dysbolism.

Meanwhile, a group given 10 g of CK-strain chlorella per day for one year showed lower blood sugar levels. Fasting blood sugar decreased from more than 250 mh/dl to 150 mg/dl; the blood sugar levels loaded with 50 g sugar were lowered from more than 350 mg/dl to 250 mh/dl. Furthermore, these patients' insulin doses decreased, from more than 10 units to five units. Their serum amino acids also decreased, ending up close to the normal value. This study shows CK-strain chlorella helps improve protein dysbolism caused by diabetes.

C. Decrease in medication dose. With diabetes, the main treatment is diet and exercise therapy, but if that isn't enough, medication is administered to control blood sugar. Recently, more patients have started using medication at relatively mild stages. Medication lowers and controls blood sugar, but it doesn't eliminate the causes of diabetes. Also, if medication isn't used with diet therapy, the appetite will intensify. Body weight and body fat will increase, causing further insulin deficiency, and blood sugar control may become more difficult.

Research shows CK-strain chlorella helps maintain blood sugar levels for patients taking blood sugar medication[11]. CVE was given for a year to a 51-year-old diabetic patient who was on a blood-sugar suppressant, with the goal of examining its effects on the levels of fasting blood sugar, triglycerides, and glycohemoglobin. After administering CVE for one year, the patient's blood sugar levels stabilized and the medication could be reduced. Glycohemoglobin, the level of which is used to test blood sugar, was lowered and became stable. This study showed that CVE is helpful for blood sugar maintenance with patients who take blood-sugar suppressants.

4. PROTECTION AGAINST ARTERIOSCLEROSIS

The saying goes, "People age as the blood vessels age." Certainly our arteries age as we grow older, but unlike naturally aged blood vessels, the abnormally aged blood vessels of arteriosclerosis are a problem. Arteriosclerosis results in heart disease and cerebrovascular disease, which cause many deaths in advanced countries.

It is crucial to discharge cholesterol from the blood and prevent abnormally aging blood vessels in order to maintain health.

CK-strain chlorella has been studied for its ability to prevent arteriosclerosis[12]. When dietary cholesterol is included in rabbit feed, serum cholesterol rises notably and sclerogenic lesions of the aortic inner membrane (in other words, arteriosclerosis) progress rapidly. Administering chlofibrate, a medication that lowers cholesterol levels, didn't deter the progress of arteriosclerosis. When CK-strain chlorella was given with dietary cholesterol, the rise in serum cholesterol was controlled, as was the progress of aortic lesions (Figure 6). This study showed that CK-strain chlorella improved abnormal conditions of serum lipids and suppressed the progress of arteriosclerosis caused by poor diet.

CK-strain chlorella helps blood vessel health by preventing cholesterol build-up and controlling the progress of arteriosclerosis. It also helps prevent heart disease and stroke.

5. PREVENTION OF STOMACH ULCERS

Our modern society is stressful, and many stress-related diseases such as stomach ulcers are on the rise. Stomach ulcers are caused by a loss of balance in the gastric juices, which digest food (the offense factor) and the protection of gastric mucin from the gastric juice (the defense factor). This means when the offense factor (excessive secretion of stomach acids and pepsin and excitement of the vagus nerves) is strong, and the defense factor (a decrease in mucus on the gastric mucin and blood flow) is lowered, gastritis and ulcers occur. Stress lowers the defense factor and strengthens the offense factor, which affects the ulcer. Recently, *Helicobacter pylori* has gotten a lot of attention as being a cause of ulcers, but this bacteria is not the only cause.

Gastric ulcers and duodenal ulcers are also called digestive ulcers. Overwork, mental stress, and irregular lifestyles are thought to cause their manifestation and recurrence.

Tests show CK-strain chlorella is effective in preventing and improving gastric ulcers[13,14]. The digestive ulcers of a rat, triggered by stress and chemicals, were prevented by the oral administration of CK-strain chlorella (Figure 7). CK-strain chlorella helps digestive

Figure 6: Effects of CK-strain on sclerogenic lesions

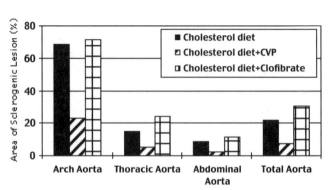

ulcers by reinforcing the defensive factor and protecting the gastric mucin.

6. PREVENTION OF ANEMIA

Blood plays an important role in transporting oxygen and nutrients throughout the body. When anemia hits, the body experiences malnutrition. Anemia can be caused by insufficient iron intake; increased iron loss through hemorrhage, parasites, heavy menstruation, or a high number of pregnancies; increased iron demand, such as that experienced in infancy, puberty, or pregnancy; and infection and malabsorption of iron.

Improvement of anemia with use of CK-strain chlorella has been studied on high school girls, pregnant women, and victims of atomic bomb blasts. Thirty female high school students who had iron-deficiency anemia were given 10 g of CK-strain chlorella per day for four months. Their hemoglobin levels, red blood cell counts, and hematocrits recovered to near normal levels[15]. Five anemic pregnant women received 2 g of CK-strain chlorella per day for three months.

Figure 7: Effect of chlorella powder and chlorella extract from CK-strain on stress-induced ulcer (by oral administration)

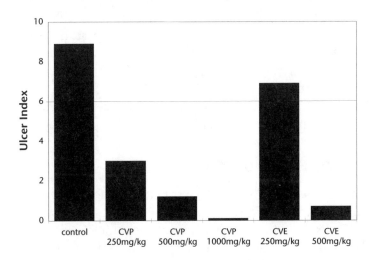

Their levels of hemoglobin and blood iron were improved[16]. Ten A-bomb victims were given 5 g of CK-strain chlorella per day for eight months, and hemoglobin and levels of red blood cells were improved[17]. CK-strain chlorella can supplement iron, which is a necessary nutrient for anemia, as well as vitamin B12 and folic acid, which aid the blood production process. Tests have shown that CK-strain chlorella is helpful for anemia.

Detoxifying Benefits of CK-strain

The human digestive system has an important job: taking in necessary nutrients for the maintenance of life. In a sense, intestines are the entrance to the body, where nutrients from food are absorbed. The intestines also serve as an entrance for toxins. If the intestines are poisoned with toxins, various diseases can result, including colon cancer, arteriosclerosis, high blood pressure, cystitis, poor skin, headaches, dizziness, stiff shoulders, stomachaches, insomnia, anorexia, hemorrhoids, allergies, and lowered immunity.

Generally, in order to detoxify, it's necessary to improve liver metabolism, including alcohol metabolism and drug metabolism; to control absorption and accelerate excretion; and to regulate the environment inside the body.

Some common toxins are dioxins, heavy metals, residual agricultural chemicals, food additives, and drugs. These materials are highly absorbable, highly residual in the body, and not easily detoxified by the liver alone.

The effect of detoxification using CK-strain chlorella is unique. It boosts not only liver metabolism, but also detoxifies those poisons that are highly residual and are not detoxified only by the liver.

1. DETOXIFICATION OF PCBS

Infection with PCBs, or polychlorinated biphenyls, began showing up in 1968 in western Japan, in Fukuoka and Nagasaki prefectures. PCBs that were used in a heating medium leaked into rice oil and caused such ailments as blackening of the skin, nails, and gums, and a rash all over the body. Later it was found that dioxin-like poisons were the cause.

Researchers have examined CK-strain chlorella's use in detoxification of PCBs[18]. Food containing 10 percent of CK-strain chlorella was fed to rats who had been injected with PCBs for four weeks. Toxic symptoms were reduced. CK-strain chlorella was also given to patients with PCB poisoning and was effective in alleviating subjective symptoms.

2. EXCRETION OF DIOXIN

Dioxin is generated in incinerators and pollutes the environment worldwide. It can also pollute our bodies when we eat food contaminated with it. Carcinogenic and generative toxicity are of most concern. Dioxin is hard to metabolize and highly residual in the body. To protect the body from damage, it is important first to avoid consuming dioxin, and then to discharge any dioxin already accumulated in the body.

CK-strain chlorella has been studied for its effects in excreting dioxin[19,20,21]. When dioxin and CK-strain chlorella were given to rats to see how absorption would be reduced, the excretion rate rose 9.8 times. CK-strain chlorella was also given to rats who had already accumulated dioxin, to learn about the acceleration of excretion, and the biological half-life of dioxin was shortened to 1/2 to 1/3. These tests show CK-strain chlorella helps inhibit absorption of dioxin and speeds up excretion of it.

3. DETOXIFICATION OF HEAVY METALS

During the 1960s, many industries expanded in Japan under the banner of economic growth. Behind the scenes, environmental pollution—Japan was even called a "pollution island"—and various health problems began appearing. The pollutants were heavy metals, and they're still damaging our health through the foods we eat.

CK-strain chlorella's usefulness in aiding detoxification of poisons triggered by pollution has been continuously studied.

A. Detoxification of cadmium. Itai-itai disease is an illness caused by cadmium poisoning. It began occurring in the 1970s along the Jintsu River in Japan's Toyama prefecture. The disease first causes kidney disorders, then osteomalacia. The illness is most aggressive in pregnant and breast-feeding women, people with endocrine irregularities, and older people with calcium deficiencies. When it becomes serious, the patient's bones break upon the slightest movement. The name of the disease came from the cries of patients, "itai-itai" ("ouch, ouch"), in response to the unbearable pain.

Tests have shown that CK-strain chlorella helps excrete cadmium[22]. After giving CK-strain chlorella to patients with cadmium poisoning, researchers noted that cadmium that had accumulated in the patients' bodies was excreted. Without the CK-strain chlorella, the cadmium was rarely excreted, but administering 6 g of CK-strain chlorella per day increased the excretion of cadmium through urine and feces.

Excretion by urine sped up metabolism of the toxins, and excretion by feces accelerated the discharge of toxins. The frequency of arthritis was also reduced, and the CK-strain chlorella improved subjective symptoms as well.

B. Detoxification of mercury. Minamata disease, caused by mercury toxicity, began showing up along the coast of Minamata Bay in Kumamoto prefecture in the 1950s and along the Agano River in Niigata prefecture in the 1960s. It's a toxic disease of the central nervous system caused by eating large amounts of fish polluted with methyl mercury for many years. The symptoms are acroagnosis, ataxia, vision reduction, and deafness.

Research has shown that CK-strain chlorella helps reduce mercury toxicity[23]. Dr. Mishima of Minamata City Hospital administered 4.5 g of CK-strain chlorella to nine patients with Minamata disease for three months. He reported that it helped alleviate malnutrition in patients with chronic organic mercury toxicity; reduced uncomfortable numbness; and increased hemoglobin, red blood cells, and serum protein.

C. Detoxification of arsenic. Blackfoot disease is an ailment that affected part of the southwest coast of Taiwan. About one hundred thousand people drank well water with 0.01 to 1.8 ppm of arsenic for more than 50 years, resulting in chronic arsenic toxicity. Symptoms of arsenic toxicity are skin cancer, keratosis, abnormal skin pigmentation, and blood vessel disorders. The illness blackens the skin so it resembles the feet of crows, hence the name blackfoot disease.

CK-strain chlorella has been studied for detoxification of arsenic[24]. When 5 g per day of CK-strain was given to patients with blackfoot disease for seven months, arsenic excretion into urine increased and arsenic levels in blood decreased, resulting in significant improvement in skin condition.

4. IMPROVEMENT OF CONSTIPATION

Due to insufficient vegetable consumption and an increase in the use of processed foods, many of us don't eat enough of the necessary nutrients for elimination, such as dietary fiber and chlorophyll. Young women especially tend to have constipation due to irregular diets.

Defecation is vital for excreting toxic substances taken in with foods. When the body is constipated, toxins stay inside the body for a long time, causing various diseases such as colon cancer, arteriosclerosis, hypertension, high blood pressure, cystitis, bad skin, headaches, dizziness, stiff shoulders, stomachaches, insomnia, anorexia, hemorrhoids, allergies, and lowered immunity. Although there are variations from individual to individual, constipation is said to exist when there are fewer than three bowel movements a week.

Tests were conducted with CK-strain chlorella on 63 female college students suffering from chronic constipation.[25] When the women were given CK-strain chlorella, their frequency of bowel movements, total amount of feces, and comfort levels were improved (Figure 8). Other conditions also improved. The treatment was effective for helping the women wake up, soothing stiff shoulders, alleviating menstrual cramps and stomachaches, and improving skin.

CK-strain chlorella contains dietary fiber, which helps ease constipation; and lipid complex and chlorophyll, which aid bowel movements by accelerating cholesterol excretion and secretion of

Figure 8A: Effects of CK-strain on constipation for female college students

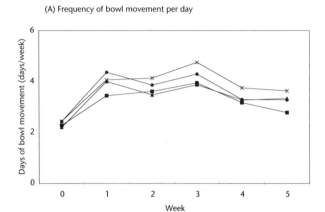

(A) Frequency of bowl movement per day

Figure 8B: Effects of CK-strain on constipation for female college students

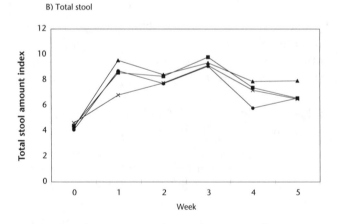

B) Total stool

bile acids. CK-strain chlorella helps improve constipation by supplementing insufficient nutrients and regulating diet balance. It also helps ease uncomfortable symptoms caused by constipation.

Immunity-Boosting Effect of CK-strain Chlorella

Our immune systems can dispose of unwanted substances, including bacteria, viruses, dead cells, cancerous cells, and virus-infected cells. Immunity is indispensable for the prevention and curing of disease. It defends the body from invaders so the body can maintain its balance. CK-strain chlorella works with this defense system to help maintain balance, promote good health, and alleviate disease.

Suppressed immunity lowers our defenses against disease. CK-strain chlorella and CVE, an active compound of CK-strain, work with the white blood cells, the main component of the immune system, to mobilize defenses and boost antiviral and antitumor function.

1. ANTITUMOR EFFECT

Cancer ranks high as a cause of death in many countries. Even with our advanced medical science, a definitive treatment for this disease has yet to be discovered. Cancer treatment currently consists of surgery, radiation, and chemotherapy. With advances in treatment, cure rates and life expectancies have improved. However, except for some types of cancer, there haven't been any satisfactory solutions for cancer recurrence and metastasis.

Deterioration of the immune system is one cause of cancer. Because of decreased immunocompetence, normal cells become malignant and multiply, causing metastasis and recurrence. To suppress the spread of cancer and reduce the side effects of treatment, it's important to boost immune function, especially of the cells in charge of immunity, such as macrophages, NK cells, and T cells.

CK-strain chlorella and CVE have been studied for treatment of tumors, boosting of immunity, suppression of metastasis, and reducing toxic conditions caused by radiation and anticancer drugs.

A. Boosting of antitumor immunity. The antitumor effect of CK-strain chlorella and CVE has been studied on mice in whom various cancer cells were artificially implanted. After oral administration of the chlorella, the study showed increased production of granulocytes and macrophages, shrinkage of tumor weight, inhibition of tumor multiplication, and prolonged life span (Figure 9).

The antitumor effect in mice injected with carrageenan, a substance derived from seaweed that is a macrophage inhibitor, has been reduced in tests. The antitumor effect of CK-strain and CVE is closely related to that of macrophages and lymphocytes. The antitumor effect is enhanced, and the inhibition of tumor multiplication is evident.

B. Inhibition of colon cancer in rats. Colon cancer is found frequently in western Europe, and it's on the rise in Japan as well. Rates of this cancer are increasing due to excessive secretion of bile acids, which is caused by high-fat diets, and a decrease in bowel movements, which is caused by low-fiber diets.

Figure 9: Tumor size reduction due to CVE administration

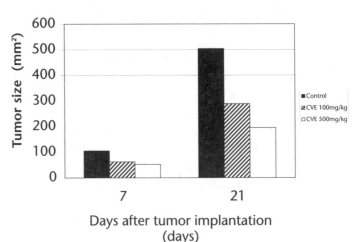

Days after tumor implantation
(days)

Hypodermic implantation of tumor cells (Meth A), 100 unit/kg, was introduced to mice. CVE was orally administered 3 days later, and the size of tumor was measured 7 and 21 days after the implantation.

CK-strain chlorella and CVE have been studied in rats with colon cancer induced by a powerful carcinogen, DMH (dimethyl-hydrazine dihydrochloride). Colon cancer in these rats was reduced by orally administering CK-strain chlorella and CVE. The manifestation rate and total number of incidences of colon cancer were reduced (Figure 10A).

When the affected cancer tissue was tested pathologically, lymphocyte infiltration was not found in the tumors of the DMH group, but significant lymphocyte infiltration was found in the CVE group (Figure 10B). This study showed CVE suppresses colon cancer induced by DMH and reduces the degree of malignancy.

C. Inhibition of tumor metastasis. Cancer metastasizes, or spreads, from the affected area to distant tissues through blood vessels in its early stages. Since this metastasized cancer is highly malignant, it makes treatment more difficult. Inhibition of cancer metastasis has become the most crucial issue in our efforts to conquer cancer.

CVE has been studied for its usefulness in suppressing cancer metastasis through testing on mice with lung cancer[31]. When cancer cells high in metastasis rate were implanted in mice, metastasized

Figure 10: Inhibition of colon cancer manifestation and amelioration in malignancy with DMH-induced rats due to CVE administration

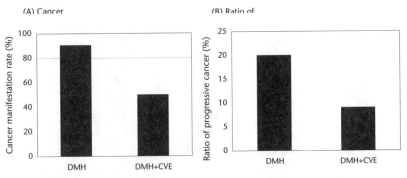

DMH (dimethyl hydrazine) 20 mg/kg was administered to rats hypodermicly once a week for 10 times. The test feeds with 1% CVE were given for 24 weeks, from the beginning of CVE administration to the end of the test. The intestinal tract was extracted and observed for the cancer manifestation rate (A) and the ratio of progressive cancer (B).

cancer cells were found in the lungs 12 days later, depending on the amount that was implanted. By administering CVE before the implantation, the metastasis amount was reduced by 1/10. By administering CVE, formation and growth of metastasized cancer cells was remarkably suppressed.

Low-metastasis-rate cancer cells, in almost all cases, didn't show any metastasis to the lungs for three weeks after implantation in normal mice. However, when cyclophosphamide, an anticancer drug, was administered two to four days before the implantation, immunity was lowered and a great deal of metastasis was found (Figure 11). And when low-metastasis-rate cancer cells were implanted after suppressing the activity of white blood cells, which fight cancer in its early stages, cancer metastasis to the lung was increased. Even with low-metastasis-rate strains, when the basic immunity function is lowered, metastasis occurs. If CVE is given under such conditions, cancer metastasized to the lungs decreases.

CVE helps prevent cancer metastasis by enhancing the function of white blood cells, which fight cancer in its early stages, and by aiding the body's ability to destroy cancer cells.

Figure 11: Effect of CVE administration on lung colony formation of B16 tumor transfer-strain(44) in CY treated mice

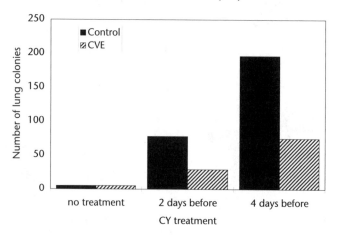

Hypodermic implantation of tumor cells (Meth A), 106 unit/kg, was introduced to mice. CVE was orally administered 3 days later, and the size of tumor was measured 7 and 21 days after the implantation.

D. Reduction of toxicity caused by radiation and anticancer drugs. Radiation and anticancer drugs are meant to kill rapidly-dividing cancer cells. But the human body contains not only cancer cells, but also normal cells that are actively dividing. Gastric mucous membranes, skin, hair roots, nails, and blood cells are examples where the side effects of radiation and anticancer drugs are conspicuous.

When white blood cells in charge of immunity decrease due to anticancer drugs, the body's resistance is lowered. This is a critical side effect of cancer treatment.

CVE works to reduce the toxicity of x-rays and anticancer drugs. When x-rays or the anticancer drug cyclophosphamide are given to rats, white blood cells of the bone marrow, spleen, and peripheral blood decrease drastically. Tests showed recovery from these symptoms is significantly accelerated by orally administering CVE continuously[32,34].

E. Improvement in function of white blood cells. CVE boosts immunity by supplementing immune cells when resistance is lowered. Research shows immune cells augmented by CVE will function better[32].

In one study, abdominal-cavity cells were treated with CVE for six to 24 hours. When these cells were implanted in normal mice together with cancer cells, the antitumor effect was evident. Even after destruction of macrophages and T cells, the antitumor activity was still there. When these cells were given to mice with immunity disorders caused by radiation, antitumor effects were not seen. When the mice were given the cells of normal mice, antitumor effects were recovered.

White blood cells that are induced by CVE show antitumor effects by some sort of activation that strengthens the immune response with the help of macrophages and T-cells. An immunity booster called OK-432 was tested the same way, but antitumor effects were not seen. This ability is one of the unique functions of CVE.

2. BOOSTING OF RESISTANCE TO INFECTION

Infectious diseases are caused by the invasion and multiplication of pathogens such as bacteria and viruses.

There are always numerous bacteria existing around us. When a bacterium enters the body, the question of whether the body will become infected depends on the body's resistance versus the virus' strength. Pathogens vary in strength, as do immune systems. When the immune system is strong, it can eliminate most bacteria, with the exception of special strains. When the immune system is weakened for some reason, even relatively feeble pathogens can cause infection. This type of infectious disease is called an opportunistic infection.

The following are some causes of lowered immunity:

• Excessive or insufficient nutrition
• Stress
• Exposure to chemical substances or intake of foods that contain them
• Medical treatment (antibiotics, radiation, anticancer drugs, and surgeries)
• Chronic diseases (metabolic disorders, such as diabetes, cirrhosis, and chronic renal failure; blood diseases, such as leukemia, lymphoma, and anemia; cancer; collagen disease; genetic immunity failure; and AIDS)

Due to such factors, opportunistic infections increase. This happens frequently in hospitals. *Staphylococcus aureus, Pseudomonas aeruginosa,* and *Escherichia coli* are examples of bacteria that cause opportunistic infections.

Antibiotics are bacteria-killing drugs; however, they only work on certain types of bacteria. Because these antibiotics are frequently used, bacteria are emerging against which antibiotics are powerless. Bacteria such as methicillin-resistant *Staphylococcus aureus* and multidrug-resisitant *Pseudomonas aeruginosa* become problematic.

The human body has the ability to fight off various bacteria. If this natural system functions properly, the body can even kill bacteria that are not affected by antibiotics. So, for the prevention of infectious disease and opportunistic infections, the immune system plays a vital role.

CVE has been studied to see if it improves immunity. Research was done by examining diseases caused by bacteria that show specific resistance to immunity. Another study looked at immune deficiency caused by anticancer drugs and lead exposure. These conditions were created to represent a state of lowered immunity.

A. Colon bacteria infection. Certain bacteria are naturally present in the large intestine. They don't become pathogens as long as they remain in the intestine, but they can cause opportunistic infection if immunity is weakened. CVE has been studied for its effects on opportunistic infection[33].

After orally administering CVE continuously for 14 days, colon bacteria were introduced into the abdominal cavity to create an infection. The number of living bacteria in the abdominal cavity, peripheral blood, spleen, and liver was counted after one hour, six hours, and 24 hours. Due to the administration of CVE, the number of bacteria in each organ was notably reduced (Figure 12A). After six hours of treating colon bacteria, high levels of multinuclear white blood cells that exuded into the abdominal cavity and peripheral blood were maintained. When the cells that exuded into the abdominal cavity were tested for bacteria-killing ability of the neutrophils, the group given CVE showed significantly higher bacteria-killing ability (Figure 12B).

The tests showed CVE helps eliminate colon bacteria by accelerating the productivity of neutrophils, which play the main role in eliminating colon bacteria, and by augmenting the ability to kill bacteria.

B. Colon bacteria infection in mice with immunity failure due to anticancer drugs. Research was conducted to find out whether CVE was helpful for boosting resistance in the case of an immunity failure. The anticancer drug cyclophosphamide was administered to mice to weaken their immunity and infect them with colon bacteria[34].

When cyclophosphamide was introduced into the abdominal cavities of mice, blood cells in the bone marrow, spleen, and

Figure 12: Effect of CVE on colon bacteria *(Escherichia coli)*

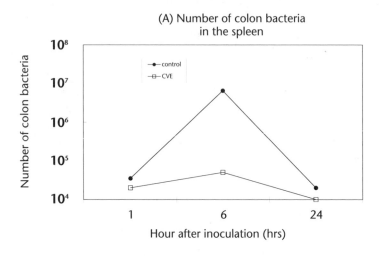

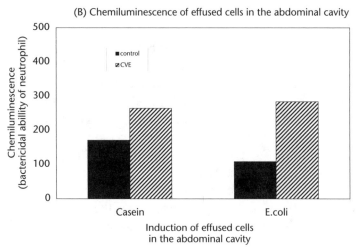

(A) Number of colon bacteria in the spleen. After orally administering CVE for 14 days, colon bacterium of 2.7~108 unit/kg body weight was implanted into the abdominal cavity. The number of colon bacteria in the spleen was measured 1, 6 and 24 hours after the introduction of infection to study the effects of CVE.

(B) Chemiluminescence of effusion cells in the abdominal cavity. After orally administering CVE for 14 days, colon bacterium (E. coli) of 2.7~108 unit/kg body weight was implanted into the abdominal cavity. Exuded cells in the abdominal cavity were collected 6 hours after the introduction of infection and chemiluminescence (bactericidal ability) of effused cells (mainly neutrophil) were studied to measure the effect of CVE.

peripheral blood became immune-deficient. Continuous oral administration of CVE alleviated the process significantly (Figure 13). Six days after cyclophosphamide treatment, colon bacteria were introduced, and the number of bacteria was significantly reduced in the CVE group. This study showed CVE improved the immunity of mice even in an immune-deficient state.

C. Listeria infection. Listeria monocytogenes resists such defense mechanisms as phagocytes and antibodies. To eliminate listeria monocytogenes, stronger immunity is required than colon bacteria. It is necessary to eliminate infected cells by boosting cellular immunity, so that abnormal cells can be destroyed through activation of macrophages and/or T-cells.

Every year 2,500 people in the United States become seriously ill with listeria, and approximately 500 people die from it. People get infected by eating contaminated foods. Symptoms include fever and muscle aches, and sometimes nausea and diarrhea. If the infection reaches the nervous system, headaches, neck stiffness, stupors, giddiness, and convulsions may occur.

CVE has been studied with listeria-infected mice for the effects on

Figure 13A: Effect of CVE administration on white blood cells of bone marrow, spleen and peripheral blood in rats

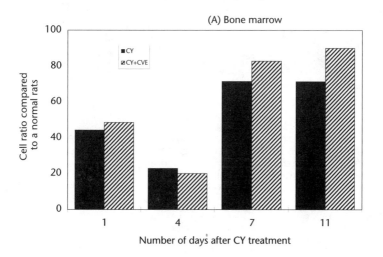

Figure 13B

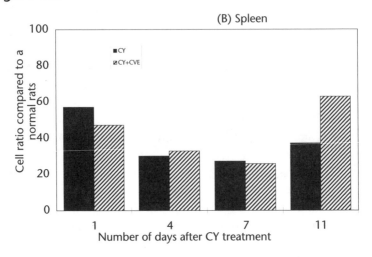

Figure 13C

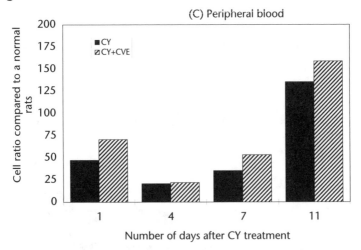

(A) After orally administering CVE for 14 days, 50mg/kg of cyclophosphamide was administered. The numbers of white blood cells of (A) bone marrow, (B) spleen and (C) peripheral blood were measured after 1,4, 7 and 11days. Each number is the ratio comparing the number of blood cells to those of a normal rat.

the hemotopoietic system response[35] (granulocyte/macrophage pro-dromic cells: CFU-GM, NK activation[36], cytokine generation[37]). When mice are infected with listeria, they die of the infection.

When CVE is orally administered to listeria-infected mice, their resistance to bacteria is enhanced by recovering granulocyte/macrophage prodromic cells (CFU-GM) (Figure 14), augmenting NK activation (Figure 15), and enforcing generation of interferonγ (IFNγ) and interleukin-2 (IL-2) (Figure 16). Research shows CVE can promote the elimination of listeria monocytogenes and prevent death caused by listeria.

D. Listeria infection in mice with immunodeficiency due to lead exposure. When mice are exposed to lead, they become immune-deficient. When the mice are infected with listeria, the function of bone marrow gets suppressed and their immunity weakens. The effects of CVE under these conditions have been studied[38].

When mice are infected with listeria, the number of CFU-GM in bone marrow decreases. Mice who were exposed to lead before they got infected with listeria had even less CFU-GM.

Figure 14: Effect of CVE administration on the hemotopoietic system of mice infected with Listeria monocytogenes

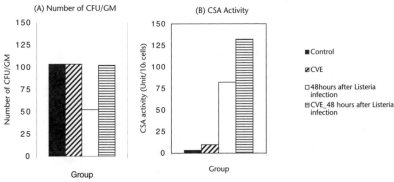

After administering CVE for 5 days, 1~10⁴unit/animal of Listeria was administered to the abdominal cavity of mice. 48 hours after being infected with Listeria, activity of the granulocyte/macrophage prodromic cells CFU-GM and CSA_serum colony stimulation activation was measured.

Figure 15: Effect of CVE administration on NK cell activity of mice infected with Listeria monocytogenes

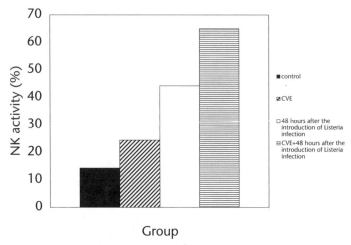

After administering CVE for 5 days, 1~10^4 unit/animal of Listeria was administered to the abdominal cavity of mice. The NK activity 48 hours after the introduction of infection was measured.

Figure 16: Effect of CVE administration on cytokine production in mice infected with Listeria monocytogenes

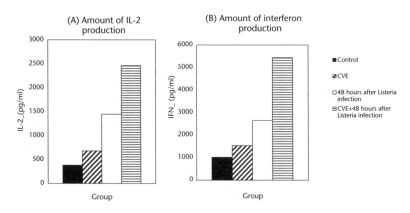

After administering CVE for 5 days, 1~10^4 unit/mouse of Listeria was administered into the abdominal cavity. The amount of IL-2 production (A) and interferon activity (B) were measured 48 hours after the introduction of infection.

When CVE is given to listeria-infected mice after lead exposure, bone marrow suppression is reduced to its normal level, and serum CSA colony stimulating activity (ability to accelerate growth and division of prodromal cells) is significantly enhanced. The thymus, an important organ of the immune system that controls the lymphocytes, loses its weight after lead exposure. However, CVE contributed to recovery of the thymus. Research shows CVE helps improve hemopoiesis of the bone marrow and resistance to listeria monocytogenes under immunodeficiency conditions.

3. ANTIALLERGY EFFECT OF CVE

The recent rise in allergic diseases such as food allergies, hay fever, and asthma has made these illnesses an important issue in advanced countries. Most patients with allergic diseases also experience allergic responses (excessive generation of IgE antibodies against allergens and abnormal augmentation of type II [Th2] helper T cells, which aid immune balance).

Helper T cells are white blood cells that control immunity. One variety is Th1, which destroys cancer cells and abnormal cells by generating γIFN (gamma-interferon) and IL-12 (interleukin-12). The other is Th2, which creates IgG and IgE antibodies by generating IL-4, IL-5, and IL-10.

Either Th1 or Th2 is activated when something in the body needs disposal. For example, when abnormal cells such as cancer cells are introduced, Th1 is augmented in order to destroy the abnormal cells. When there is something that needs to be cleaned out of the blood, such as an influenza virus, Th2 is boosted to generate antibodies. The theory goes that in allergy diseases, Th2 alone is abnormally augmented, so the ability to make antibodies is excessively sensitive.

It has traditionally been very difficult to analyze food allergies. The reason is, while an allergen from the mouth establishes immune tolerance, successive allergic responses supposedly coming after the tolerance (excessive IgE antibody generation against the allergen and abnormal augmentation of Th2) don't occur.

Professor Yoshikai of Nagoya University successfully developed the food allergy animal model, in which the IgE antibodies are boosted by administering milk casein food to DBA/2 mice[39]. The development of this model made it possible to analyze the mechanism of food allergy.

CVE has been studied with this food allergy model for its antiallergic effect[40]. When milk casein is given to DBA/2 mice, IgE antibodies are augmented in the blood against milk casein to create food allergies. When CVE was orally administered to mice with this allergic condition, IgE generation against milk casein was suppressed (Figure 17). Also, mRNA in γIFN, IL-12, and Th1 were augmented.

In allergic diseases, Th2 becomes dominant and abnormal generation of antibodies occurs. Research shows CVE sedates the generation of abnormal antibodies by balancing helper T cells. In this way, CVE helps prevent and alleviate allergy diseases.

Figure 17: Inhibition of IgE production against milk casein by CVE administration

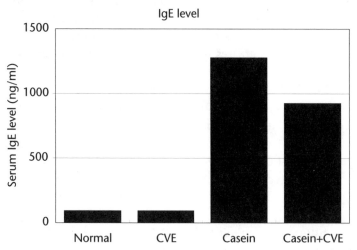

Feeds with 20% casein and 2% CVE were given to mice for 2 weeks and IgE levels against casein in the serum were measured.

4. ANTIVIRUS EFFECT OF CVE

A virus is a living organism that invades specific cells of the body and multiplies using the metabolism system of the cells, causing weakened immunity. Some viral diseases are AIDS, hepatitis B and C, herpes, and influenza. Viruses and bacteria each require different types of immunity. A virus in the blood can be killed by marshaling antibodies. For viral infections in organs and systems, boosting immune function is necessary in order to destroy abnormal cells infected by the virus. CVE has been studied with cytomegalovirus and the AIDS virus for antivirus effect.

A. Cytomegalovirus infection. Cytomegalovirus is a global phenomenon. By the age of 40, 50 to 80 percent of the U.S. population has been infected.

If pregnant women are infected with cytomegalovirus and the fetuses get infected, about 10 percent of babies may show some type of abnormality. Premature birth, swollen liver and spleen, rashes, cerebral ventricle calcification around the brain, retinitis, and pneumonia may occur. Children who are born with one of these abnormalities are more likely to have deafness, retardation, or vision problems. Even if there is no apparent abnormality at birth, 10 percent may have some kind of nerve disorder later. When healthy people are infected, there are generally no symptoms.

CVE has been studied in mice with cytomegalovirus (MCMV) for its antivirus effect[41]. When a lethal dose of MCMV was given to mice in one study, all the mice died. All the mice given CVE survived. When the virus-infected spleens and livers of the mice that were fed CVE were studied, the virus multiplication was inhibited in those organs, and tissue damage was also prevented (Figure 18A). Interferon production (Figure 18B), 2-5A synthetic enzyme activity, and NK activity (Figure 18C) were also enhanced.

CVE provides antivirus protection by improving NK activity in order to destroy infected cells and by augmenting interferon activity in serum.

B. MAIDS virus infection. AIDS is a viral disease caused by HIV (human immunodeficiency virus) infection. Once infected, the

Figure 18: Effect of CVE on Murine cytomegalovirus infection

(A) Number of viruses in the organs

(B) Amount of interferon production

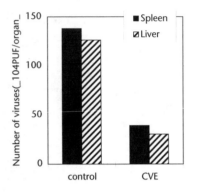

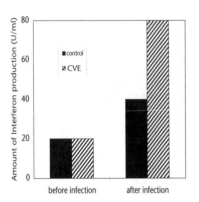

(C) NK activity

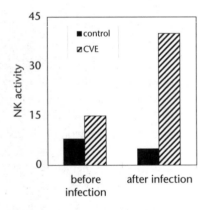

1 or 3 day after implanting cytomegalovirus, CVE was administered. 1~10⁶ PFU of cytomegalovirus was implanted, and the number of viruses in organs (A), amount of interferon production (B) and NK activity (C) were measured.

immune system is destroyed and resistance is weakened, giving rise to various infectious diseases and malignant tumors.

CVE has been studied for its effects using the MAIDS virus (LP-BM5), which is the pathological model of AIDS. When mice are infected with MAIDS, just as in humans, their immune systems fail and they become vulnerable to bacterial infections. When CVE was orally administered about two weeks after the MAIDS virus was introduced, the infection resistance against bacteria was boosted.

CVE administration improves helper T cell function and supports killer T cells. Studies show that the decrease of Thy1.2$^+\alpha\beta^+$T cells (T cells that kill abnormal cells in early formation) was prevented within four weeks after introduction of the infection[42].

These tests showed CVE improved the function of immune cells damaged by the MAIDS virus and supported specific cellular immunity against bacteria. To analyze the role of CVE in relation to MAIDS, the gene expressions of cytokine (IL-1α, TNF, GM-CSF, IL-12, γIFN, and IL-10), which are secreted by cells that are in charge of immunity, have been studied[43].

After orally administering CVE to normal mice for two weeks and collecting abdominal-cavity cells, cytokine gene expressions, which are vital for cellular immunity, were boosted at the genetic level (Figure 19). After orally administering CVE to normal mice and MAIDS mice for two weeks, listeria was introduced into the abdominal cavity. Six days after the introduction, gene expressions

Figure 19: Amount of cytokine gene production in normal mice administered CVE

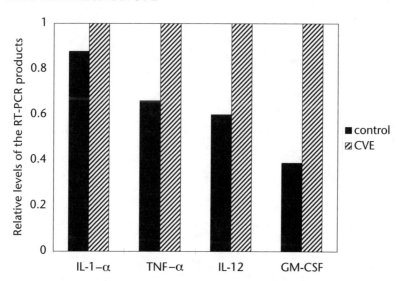

After orally administering CVE to normal mice for 2 weeks, effused cells in the abdominal cavity (macrophage compartment) were collected, and the cytokine gene manifestation was investigated by RCR method.

of γIFN and IL-12 were augmented and expressions of IL-10 were decreased (Figure 20).

CVE approaches the macrophages first, then accelerates creation of inflammatory cytokine (IL-1α, TNF-α) and IL-12. CVE improved defense by augmenting cellular immunity using γIFN, IL-12 generated by NK cells, and macrophages. Even in an immune-deficient state due to virus infection, CVE enhances immunity to help eliminate virus and bacteria.

Figure 20: Cytokine production in a normal mouse, MAIDS mouse and Listeria infected mouse.

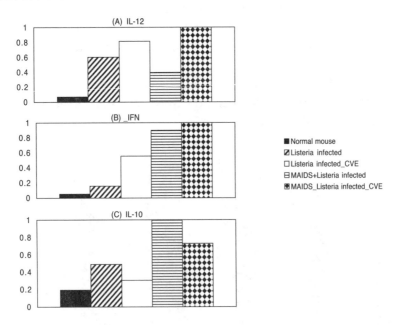

Leukemia virus LP-BM5 MuLV was introduced into the abdominal cavity and 2x104 units of L.monocytogenes were administered into the abdominal cavity 4 weeks later. Feeds with 2% CVE were administered 2 weeks after LP-BM5 was introduced and continued after introduction of Listeria infection, as well. Cytokine genes were investigated in the spleen 6 days after the introduction of Listeria infection.

Activation of cells by CK-strain Chlorella

The human body consists of approximately 60 trillion cells. Each of these cells generates energy that we need in order to survive. For example, the heart works continuously for 24 hours a day through energy generated by each cell. If energy isn't being created, the function of the cardiac muscle will decrease and symptoms such as shortness of breath and palpitation will occur.

Each cell works to generate energy through the food we eat. Unless the required nutrition is properly supplemented and burned, cells cannot generate energy, and we die. Our bodies are constantly exchanging old cells for new cells, a process known as metabolism. Metabolism is indispensable for sustaining life, and a lowered metabolism can cause poor health. The body's energy is created by cell metabolism.

1. MITOCHONDRIA GENERATE ENERGY

Energy is created when oxygen burns nutrients in small organelles inside cells called mitochondria. One cell contains approximately 50 to 100 mitochondria.

Ninety-five percent of the body's energy is produced by these little powerhouses. The more an organ requires energy metabolism—such as skeletal muscles, the heart, liver, kidneys, and brain—the more mitochondria are found. That's why the heart can operate continuously with abundant energy.

When energy production deteriorates, our activities are affected in many ways. If our muscle strength is weakened, it's easy for us to trip on an object. If the cardiac muscle gets weak, we'll have shortness of breath. If the liver is weakened, we'll get drunk fast when consuming alcohol, even if this wasn't the case when we were younger. One of the major causes of all these symptoms is weakened energy production.

To avoid these symptoms, we must maintain and improve our energy production.

2. CAUSES OF ENERGY SHORTAGE

When we are in poor physical condition and get sick, we feel listless or fatigued. These are subjective symptoms because our bodies have an energy shortage. The following are some causes of energy shortage:

A. Nutrition deficiency. Some diets don't supply the nutrients necessary to generate energy. Taking in enough vitamins and minerals is crucial to energy production.

B. Decreased blood flow. Oxygen shortage is our worst natural enemy. Oxygen shortage decreases the efficiency of energy generation and causes accumulation of lactic acid, which causes fatigue.

C. Mineral imbalance. When the body moves and sweats, water and electrolytes (minerals) are lost. Shortages of minerals such as magnesium and calcium cause imbalance and fatigue in the body.

D. Malfunction of brain regulation. Continuous mental work causes fatigue that results in sluggish sending and receiving of information in the brain. Efficiency decreases after doing continuous simple calculations because the information exchange becomes stagnant in the brain, causing mental tiredness.

3. HOW CVE IMPROVES ENERGY PRODUCTION

To produce energy, we must supplement the food we eat and improve blood flow. CK-strain chlorella sets an environment for energy production by supplementing vitamins and minerals, which aid energy production, and by improving blood flow due to its cleansing effect on the blood and blood vessels and its detoxification abilities.

CVE also speeds up the formation of mitochondria, the body's energy factories,[44,45] which accelerates the synthesis of energy and improves physical functioning. CK-strain's cellular activating effect, mentioned earlier, is a typical example.

Energy is used wherever sustenance of life is necessary. Therefore, when energy is deficient, it's impossible to maintain health, much less improve it.

How to Use Chlorella

Chlorella products are available in the form of tablets, powders, and liquids. The following describes how to take tablets and powders.

For regular use, 2 to 3g of chlorella is recommended per day. For people with active lifestyles, the dosage may be increased to 4 to 10g per day. For those who have health concerns and want to improve their health, 4 to 10g is recommended. You may want to consult your health professional for further advice.

Chlorella may be taken with any liquid—water, juice, coffee, tea, soup—after meals. Anybody, including children and seniors, can use it.

If you're taking other health food supplements or medication, chlorella can be added to your regimen. The only thing to avoid when taking chlorella is the medication Coumadin (warfarin sodium). Coumadin is used for people who have had cardiac valve implants, and it affects anticoagulation and antithrombosis by inhibiting the synthesis of vitamin K-dependent blood coagulation factor in the liver. Chlorella is rich in vitamin K, so it is not recommended for those who take Coumadin.

Conclusion

We've explained that CK-strain chlorella's nutritional value lies in its high-quality plant protein, vitamins, minerals, and chlorophyll. We've outlined its many benefits: cleansing the blood by eliminating excess cholesterol; suppressing high blood pressure; improving diabetes; preventing arteriosclerosis by making blood vessels more flexible; alleviating stomach ulcers; detoxification; regulating the intestines; and boosting immune function.

Poor diet causes various diseases. Supplements such as chlorella can fill the gaps created by foods low in nutrition and enhance your natural healing power by stimulating the systems that maintain the body's balance. Adding CK-strain chlorella to your diet can help you achieve vibrant health.

References

1. Mitsuda, H., Nishikawa, Y., Higuchi, M., Nakajima, K., and Kawai, F.: Effect of the breaking of chlorella cells on the digestibility of chlorella protein. J.Jpn.Soc.Nutr.Food Sci 30 (2), 93-98 (1977).

2. Komaki, H., Yamashita, M., Niwa, Y., Tanaka, Y., Kamiya, N., Ando, Y., and Furuse, M.: The effect of processing of chlorella vulgaris ck-5 on in vitro and in vivo digestibility in rats. Animal Feed Science and Technology 70, 363-366 (1998).

3. Sanno, T.: The effect of chlorella on alimentary hyperlipemia in rats: the localization and mechanisms of hypolipemic activity in chlorella. J. Kurume Med. Assoc 45(11), 1130-1153 (1982).

4. Fujiwara, Y., Hirakawa, K. , Shinpo, K.: Effect of long-term administration of chlorella tablets on hyperlipemia. J.Jpn.Soc.Nutr.Food Sci 43(3), 167-173 (1990).

5. Suzuki, T., et al. Effects of digested products from several protein food sources on blood pressure in hypertensive rats. Japan Heart J. 20, 337-339(1979).

6. Hasegawa, T.: The effect of lowering blood pressure by oral administration of chlorella on spontaneous hypertension in rats. Chlorella Industry Co., LTD. Annual Report 4, 226-227 (1983).

7. Miyawaki, M.: Research of chlorella (Chikugo strain) No. 4—About Hypertension—Chlorella Industry Co., LTD. Annual Report 4, 59-68 (1983).

8. Tokuyasu, M., Hashikawa, A.: Study of chlorella, effects on diabetes control. General meeting of the Japanese Society of Nutrition and Dietetics (1990).

9. Tokuyasu, M., Hashikawa, A.: Effect of administration of chlorella on elderly patients with complications caused by diabetes (No. 2). General meeting of the Japanese Society of Nutrition and Dietetics (1994).

10. Fukui, S.: Study on amino acid metabolism with patients with urinary diseases. Chlorella Industry Co., LTD. Annual Report 3, 95-106 (1979).

11. Unpublished data.

12. Sanno, T., Watanabe, K., Kumamoto, Y., Okuda, M., and Tanaka, Y.: The effects of chlorella on experimental atherosclerosis in rabbits. J.Jpn. Atherosclerosis Sci. 8(1), 219-225 (1980).

13. Tanaka, K., Maruyama, I., and Kanno, T.: Oral administration of a unicellular green algae, chlorella vulgaris, prevents stress-induced ulcer. Chlorella Industry Co., LTD. Annual Report 10, 13-21 (2000).

14. Tanaka, K., Yamada, A., Noda, K., Shyoama ,Y., Kubo, C., and Nomoto, K.: Oral administration of a unicellular green algae, chlorella vulgaris, prevents stress-induced ulcer. Planta Medica 63, 465-466 (1997).

15. Tokuyasui, M., Fujiwara, Y.: Discussion on the use of chlorella in anemia diet therapy for female high school students. General meeting of the Japanese Society of Nutrition and Dietetics (1978).

16. Sonoda, M.: Effects of chlorella on pregnant women. The Japanese Society of Nutrition and Dietetics, 30(5), 30-37 (1972).

17. Sonoda, M.: Changes in red blood cells, white blood cells, and hemoglobin due to long-term use of chlorella. Chlorella Industry Co., LTD. Annual Report 7, 179-183 (1990).

18. Hoshide, M., Nakajima, Y., Yagi, K., Amano, M., Okuda, T., Umeda, G., Tanaka, Y., Okuda, M., and Hasegawa, T.: PCB study of therapeutic and preventive effects of chlorella preparation on the intoxication process. General meeting of Japan Society for Occupational Health (1974).

19. Morita, K., Matsueda, T., and Iida, T.: Effect of chlorella, spirulina, and chlorophyllin on fecal excretion of polychlorinated dibenzo-p-dioxins in rats. J.Toxicol.Environ.Health. 43(3), 167-173 (1997).

20. Morita, K., Matsueda, T., Iida, T., and Hasegawa, T.: Chlorella accelerates dioxin excretion in rats. Journal of Nutrition 129(9), 1731-1736 (1999).

21. Morita, K., Ogata, M., and Hasegawa, T.: Chlorophyll derived from chlorella inhibition dioxin absorption from the gastrointestinal tract and accelerates dioxin excretion in rats. Environmental Health Perspectives 109(3), 289-294 (2001).
22. Ichimura, S.: Effect of chlorella on urine and fecal excretion of cadmium in itai-itai disease patients. General meeting of the Pharmaceutical Society of Japan (1973).
23. Mishima, I., Kuwano, R.: The case for grosmin administration for chronic Minamata disease patients. Unpublished data.
24. Itimura, S.: Effect of chlorella administration for treating blackfoot disease in the southern coast of Taiwan. General meeting of Japanese Society for Hygiene (1975).
25. Fujiwara, Y., Shinpo, K., Imae, Y., Nonomura, M., and Hirakawa, K.: Effect of chlorella vulgaris strain CK-5 on the frequency of bowel movement in humans. Jpn.J.Nutr.Diet. 56(5),253-263(1998).
26. Tanaka, K., Konishi, F., Nomoto, K., Ueno, S., Ueno, K., Sano, T., and Okuda, M.: Effects of the oral administration of unicellular algae, chlorella vulgaris, for antitumor and its mechanism. Chlorella Industry Co., LTD. Annual Report 5, 50-55 (1986).
27. Justo, G.Z., Silva, M.R., and Queiroz, M.L.S.: Effects of the green algae chlorella vulgaris on the response of the host hematopoietic system to intraperitoneal Ehrlich ascites tumor transplantation in mice. Immunopharmacol. Immunotoxicol. 23(1), 119-132 (2001).
28. Tanaka, K., Tomita, Y., Tsuruta, M., Konishi, F., Okuda, M., Himeno, K., and Nomoto, K.: Oral administration of chlorella vulgaris augments concomitant antitumor immunity. Immunophamacol.Immunotoxicol. 12(2) 277-291 (1990).
29. Konishi, F., Kanno, T., Kumamoto, Y., Hasegawa, T., and Kumamoto, S.: Effects of oral administration of chlorella vulgaris CK-5 strain extract for suppressing cancer in rats. General meeting of the Japanese Society for Complementary and Alternative Medicine (2003).
30. Kumamoto, Y., Sanno, T., Ueno, K., Hasegawa, T., Okuda, M., and Tanaka, Y.: DMH effects of chlorella on inhibiting colon cancer of induced rats. General meeting of the Japan Society for Bioscience, Biotechnology, and Agrochemistry (1985).
31. Konishi, F., Ueno, S., Kanno, T., Hasegawa, T., Kumamoto, S.,

Amdo, Y., and Nomoto, K.: Effects of chlorella vulgaris CK-5 extract (CVE) for suppressing lung transfer tumors in rats. General meeting of the Japanese Society for Complementary and Alternative Medicine (2002).

32. Konishi, F.: Augmentation of host defense mechanisms by unicellular green algae, chlorella vulgaris: resistance to meth A tumor and escherichia coli infection. Journal of the Osaka City Medical Center 38, (3), 469-484 (1989).

33. Hasegawa, T., Tanaka, K., Ueno, K., Ueno, S., Okuda, M., Yoshikai, Y., and Nomoto, K.: Augmentation of the resistance against escherichia coli by oral administration of hot water extract of chlorella vulgaris in rats. Int.J.Immunopharmac. 11, (8), 971-976 (1989).

34. Hasegawa, T., Yoshikai, Y., Okuda, M., and Nomoto, K.: Accelerated restoration of the leukocyte number and augmented resistance against escherichia coli in cyclophosphamide-treated rats orally administered with a hot water extract of chlorella vulgaris. Int.J.Immunopharmac., 12, (8), 883-891 (1990).

35. Dantas, D.C.M., Queiroz, M.L.S: Effects of chlorella vulgaris on bone marrow progenitor cell of mice infected with listeria monocytogenes. Int.J.Immunopharmacol. 21, 499-508 (1999).

36. Dantas, D.C.M., Kaneno, R., and Queiroz, M.L.S.: Effects of chlorella vulgaris in the protection of mice infected with listeria monocytogenes. Role of natural killer cells. Int. J.Immunopharmacol. 21, 609-619 (1999).

37. Queiroz, M.L.S., Bincoletto, C., Valadared, M.S., Dantas, D.V.M., and Santos, L.M.B.: Effects of chlorella vulgaris extract on cytokines production in listeria monocytogenes-infected mice. Immunopharmacol.Immunotoxical. 24, (3), 483-496 (2002).

38. Queiroz, M.L.S., Rodrigues, A.P.O., Bincoletto, C., Figueiredo, C.A.V., and Malacrida, S.: Protective effects of chlorella vulgaris in lead-exposed mice infected with listeria monocytogenes. Int. Immunopharmmacl. 3, 889-900 (2003).

39. Yoshikai, Y.: Murine model of production with a predominant Th2 response by feeding protein without adjuvants. Chlorella Industry Co., LTD. Annual Report 11, 84-91 (2003).

40. Hasegawa, T., Ito, K., Ueno, S., Kumamoto, S., Ando, Y., Yamada, A., Nomoto, K., and Yoshikai, Y.: Oral administration of hot water extracts of chlorella vulgaris reduces IgE production against milk

casein in mice. Int.J.Immunopharmacol. 21, 311-323 (1999).
41. Ibusuki, K., Minamishima, Y.: Effect of chlorella vulgaris extract on murine cytomegalovirus infection. Natural Immunity and Cell Growth Regulation 9, 121-128 (1990).
42. Hasegawa, T., Okuda, M., Makino, M., Hirommatsu, K., Nomoto, K., and Yoshikai, T.: Hot water extracts of chlorella vulgaris reduce opportunistic infection with listeria monocytogenes in C57BL/6 mice infected with LP-BM5 murine leukemia viruses. Int.J.Immunopharmacol. 17, (6), 505-512 (1995).
43. Hasegawa, T., Kimura, Y., Hirommatsu, K., Kobayashi, N., Yamada, A., Makino, M., Okuda, M., Sano, T., Nomoto, K., and Yoshikai, T.: Effect of hot water extracts of chlorella vulgaris on cytokine expression patterns in mice with murine acquired immunodeficiency syndrome after infection with listeria monocytogenes. Immunopharmacol. 35, 273-282 (1997).
44. Okuda, M.: Biological action of chlorella extract (3): preventive effect on induction of RD mutation and acceleration of cytochrome biosynthesis in yeast. J.Med.Soc.Toho,Japan 18(5), 743-750 (1971).
45. Okuda, M., Takada, H.: Effect of extract of light-grown chlorella cells on the induction of respiratory-deficient mutant of yeast by cationic surfactant. Boukinboubai 3(4), 160-165 (1975).

About the Author

Toshihiro Kanno, Ph.D. was graduated from Department of Pharmacology at Kitasato University, then he received Ph.D. degree from Faculty of Natural Science at Chiba University. He is one of well-known living chlorella specialists, and is also a pharmacist as well as a functional food advisor licensed from Japan Health Food & Nutrition Food Association. (www.jhnfa.org/hoken2.html)

Toshi is a well-known educator of functional foods, especially chlorella vulgaris (Chikugo strain with CVE: more than 500 research studies done since 1964) in Japan and the U.S. He educates pharmacists and health conscious consumers, and is currently giving holistic lectures throughout Japan and the U.S. speaking of the importance of staying healthy in anti-aging perspective. His down-to-earth health talk to consumers is well understood and accepted without complicated medical and biological terminologies.

Toshi's doctoral dissertation was "In search of functional properties of chlorella vulgaris" and currently participates in many chlorella studies. His treatise in 1997 "Functional properties of chlorella vulgaris" is well respected in the industry.

Woodland Health Series

Definitive Natural Health Information At Your Fingertips!

The Woodland Health Series offers a comprehensive array of single topic booklets, covering subjects from fibromyalgia to green tea to acupressure. If you enjoyed this title, look for other WHS titles at your local health-food store, or contact us. Complete and mail (or fax) us the coupon below and receive the complete Woodland catalog and order form—free!

Or . . .

- Call us toll-free at (800) 777-2665
- Visit our Web site
  (www.woodlandpublishing.com)
- Fax the coupon (and other correspondence) to
  (801) 334-1913

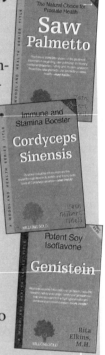

Woodland Publishing Customer Service

448 EAST 800 NORTH • OREM, UTAH • 84097

❑ *YES! Send me a free Woodland Publishing catalog.*
❑ *YES! Send me a free issue of the* WOODLAND HEALTH REPORT *newsletter.*

Name _____

Address _____

_____

_____

City _____ State _____ Zip Code _____

Phone _____ email _____